Contents

INTRODUCTION

It's hard to see a loved one hurting. Caring for a person in pain can leave you feeling tired and discouraged. To keep from feeling overwhelmed, you might consider asking other family members and friends for help. Or, some community service organizations might offer short-term, or respite, care. worryless with cbd oil can help treat numerous forms of pain in a wide variety of patients, including back pain, cancer pain, fibromyalgia pain, arthritis, and migraines. Up until recently, patient's were relying on anecdotal evidence. Now, these clinical trials into the benefits of CBD oil are proving positive.

Dealing with chronic pain can be disruptive to your life in many ways. While aches and pains are a pretty normal part of life, it can seem pretty damaging mentally and physically when it happens every day. If you have ever felt this way, you most likely have already sought out other options. The problem is, most doctors want to throw a pill at the problem. When you get on medications, they most likely have a long list of terrifying side effects including death. At that point, you would rather deal with the pain.

The CBD Oil for Pain Relief: offers a comprehensive guide for how much CBD oil to take based on your weight and pain level, which brands of CBD oil to purchase, and how not to lose money in a new and booming industry. It addresses the "legality" issue, and gives you recipes for pain-relieving salves and moisturizers, which include CBD oil as a main ingredient.

Don't wait another moment to change your life, rid yourself of crippling medications, and seek a natural cure to your pain via CBD oil?

CBD

CBD stands for cannabidiol. It is one of 113 cannabinoids that's found in cannabis. It is non-addictive and also non-psychoactive. CBD is extracted from the cannabis plant during production and is separated from the THC, which is the psychoactive element of cannabis. Cannabidiol (CBD) is one of many cannabinoids that can be found in hemp and marijuana, two types of cannabis plants.

CBD may help people with cancer manage some symptoms of the disease as well as side effects of treatment. Scientists are also looking into how CBD could aid cancer treatment, but more research is needed before any conclusions can be made.

Marijuana has enough tetrahydrocannabinol (THC) to get you high, but hemp does not. CBD itself has no psychoactive compounds

CBD oil has garnered a reputation as being an effective treatment for neurological and physiological illnesses. People who use CBD oil love that it's a natural product that is generally much easier on the body when compared to most pharmaceuticals. It's commonly used to treat pain, anxiety, and insomnia, but can CBD oil work for cancer patients?

Those that want to seek the supposed relief that cannabis may provide, may now seek it through the use of CBD. Those suffering from anxiety, depression, pain, cancer, and other ailments are turning to CBD for the possible relief and bodily equilibrium that it may provide. There are not any known health risks associated with CBD… however; those taking certain medication should proceed with caution. In any case, we recommend consulting with a medical professional for those who take medication which may interact with grapefruit (Read more about CBD drug interactions here. In fact, there are innumerable reports throughout common widespread media that attribute CBD to its' positive prophylactic effects

This book will take an in-depth look at everything you need to know about using CBD for cancer treatment.

How Are CBD Products Made?

Many people know that CBD comes from cannabis. It's right there in the name: cannabidiol.

But, how exactly does CBD oil get made? What happens in the transition from the hemp plant to a product you can buy online or in your local health store?

All CBD products contain CBD oil, which is extracted from the hemp plant. This is why you'll often see "hemp extract" on the label and in the ingredients list. After extraction, the oil is added to various products, including CBD oil tinctures, gummies, capsules, topicals, and vape oils.

CBD Extraction Methods

When people talk about how CBD products are made, they're mainly talking about the specific extraction method. The most common methods to extract CBD oil use carbon dioxide, steam distillation, or hydrocarbon or natural solvents. We review each of these below.

Carbon Dioxide (CO2) Extraction

CO2 extraction uses supercritical carbon dioxide to separate the CBD oil from the plant material. "Supercritical" refers to the CO2 containing properties of both a liquid and a gas state, which is why you'll sometimes see this method referred to as Supercritical Fluid Extraction (SFE).

During CO2 extraction, a series of pressurized chambers and pumps are used to expose CO2 to high pressure and very low temperatures, resulting in an extracted oil containing high amounts of CBD.

At the start of extraction, one chamber will hold pressurized CO_2, while a second pressurized chamber holds the hemp plant.

The CO_2 is then pumped from the first chamber into the second. The presence of supercritical CO_2 breaks down the hemp also in the chamber, causing the oil to separate from the plant material.

Finally, the CO_2 and oil are pumped together into a third chamber. The gas evaporates, leaving an extract of pure CBD oil behind.

While it requires expensive specialized machinery, CO_2 extraction is the preferred method for making CBD products. It's extremely safe and efficient at producing high concentrations of CBD in the resulting oil—as much as 92% according to one analysis.

Carbon dioxide extraction for CBD oil

The precise nature of CO2 extraction also makes it suitable for producing specific concentrations of CBD oil. Manufacturers can simply adjust the solvent and pressure ratios to achieve the desired concentration of CBD.

The CO2 extraction process is also widely used to create many other products besides CBD oil, such as decaffeinating coffee or tea, or extracting essential oils for use in perfumes.

Steam Distillation

With steam distillation, steam causes the CBD oil to separate from the hemp plant.

The hemp plant is contained in a glass flask, with an inlet and an outlet. The inlet connects to another glass container, beneath the plant flask, that contains water that is set to boil. The outlet connects to a condenser tube.

Steam distillation for cbd

As the water heats up, the steam travels upwards into the plant flask, separating the oil vapors that contain CBD.

These vapors are then captured in a tube that condenses them into oil and water.

Once collected, the oil and water mixture is distilled to extract the CBD oil from the water.

The steam distillation technique is tried and true, having been used to extract essential oil for centuries, but it's less preferred than CO_2 extraction due to its inefficiency. Steam distillation requires significantly larger amounts of hemp plant, and it's more difficult to extract exact amounts of CBD concentration using this method.

There's also an element of risk with this method. If the steam gets too hot, it can damage the extract and alter the chemical properties of the cannabinoids it contains.

Solvent Extraction (Hydrocarbons and Natural Solvents)

Solvent extraction follows a similar process to steam distillation, except that it uses a solvent rather than water to separate the CBD oil from the plant material. This creates a resulting mixture of the CBD oil with the solvent. The solvent then evaporates leaving pure CBD oil behind. Solvent extraction uses either hydrocarbons or natural solvents.

Solvent extraction is more efficient than steam distillation, and it's also less expensive. However, the solvents used in hydrocarbon extraction (including naphtha, petroleum, butane, or propane) create cause for concern. The solvent residue can be toxic and increase one's cancer risk if they aren't fully eliminated during the evaporation step—which doesn't always happen. Some studies have found traces of petroleum or naphtha hydrocarbons residue in CBD products that used solvent extraction.

To avoid the risk of toxic residue, solvent extraction can use natural solvents instead, such as olive oil or ethanol. These solvents are just as effective at extracting CBD oil, but remove the risk of toxic residue.

However, natural solvent extraction is not without its downsides. When natural solvents like ethanol are used, chlorophyll may also be extracted. This gives the resulting oil an unpleasant taste. If the CBD is used in capsules or topicals, this isn't a big deal, but many CBD products are eaten or inhaled (such as gummies, tinctures, vape oils), so this can make them harder to sell.

The larger problem with natural solvents, though, is that they don't evaporate very well. As a result, the CBD extract contains a lower concentration of CBD than it would with other methods.

What Is the Best Extraction Method for CBD Oil?

There are pros and cons to each extraction method. At CBDOil.org, we recommend CO_2 extraction. While it is the most expensive extraction method, it consistently produces the highest concentration of CBD, resulting in a quality product. It's also one of the safest extraction methods, leaving behind no neurotoxic residue.

Extraction Method Pros Cons

CO2 Extraction Efficient

Highest concentration of CBD

Easier to adjust concentration

No toxic residue

No chlorophyll Expensive

Steam Distillation Inexpensive

No toxic residue

No chlorophyll Inefficient

Inconsistent concentration of CBD

Potential for heat to damage CBD oil

Hydrocarbon Solvent Extraction Efficient

Inexpensive

Consistent concentration of CBD

No chlorophyll Potential for toxic solvent residue

Natural Solvent Extraction Efficient

Inexpensive

No toxic residue Presence of chlorophyll affects taste

Lower concentration of CBD

When purchasing CBD products, find out which extraction method the company uses, as this can be an indicator of the quality and value of their products. Products that use CO2 extraction may be more expensive, but they also tend to be higher-quality.

CBD products made using other extraction methods can be safe and high-quality as well, but there can be more risk with these products. Specifically, CBD products that were made using hydrocarbon extraction may contain solvent residuals. And while steam distillation and natural solvent extraction are lower-risk, they can produce lower or inconsistent amounts of CBD, which can affect the cost/mg value of your CBD product.

Beyond their extraction method, also confirm that the company uses a third-party lab to test the concentration of the CBD in their products, as well as the safety of the other ingredients. Any reputable manufacturer will make these test results readily available on their website, with their product packaging, or upon request. The test results will show the potency of the CBD and other cannabinoids (described in milligrams). They'll also reveal any potential contaminants, as well as the presence of any solvent residue, if the product used hydrocarbon solvent extraction.

What Happens After Extraction?

After extraction, the resulting CBD oil is described as "full-spectrum." This means that other cannabinoids besides CBD, including CBDA, CBDV, THC, and others, are still present. As long as the product is sourced from hemp, the amount of THC will be 0.3% or less (which makes it legal anywhere in the U.S.).

Full-spectrum CBD oils also contain other beneficial elements from the plant material, such as terpenes and amino acids. Many people prefer full-spectrum CBD oil because of the "entourage effect." While this effect has not been proven, some users believe that the CBD is able to engage the endocannabinoid system more effectively when more cannabinoids are present.

However, some people would rather have no THC in their oil, even in very low, legal amounts. These people prefer CBD isolates. To create CBD isolate, the extract is cooled and further purified into crystalline isolate form. This results in a white, flavorless powder. Because it contains only CBD, CBD isolate is less expensive per milligram, contains no THC, and has no flavor or odor.

Finally, regardless of whether it is turned into a CBD isolate or remains full-spectrum, the CBD oil is added to other substances to create various CBD products.

The CBD may be mixed with a carrier oil like hemp seed oil or coconut oil to create CBD oil tinctures.

To create CBD gummies, the CBD oil may be combined with natural flavoring, juice, and organic corn syrup.

The CBD oil may be mixed with a variety of ingredients to create CBD edibles like baked goods or chocolates.

With CBD capsules, the CBD oil is often added to MCT oil (a coconut oil extract) to give the capsule volume. If it's a softgel, the capsule may also use olive oil to create the casing.

To create CBD vape oils, the CBD oil is combined with a mix of vegetable glycerin and propylene glycol (to make it suitable for inhalation) and natural flavoring (for better taste).

The CBD oil may be combined with various essential oils, shea butter, aloe vera, and waxes to create CBD creams, skin salves, and other topicals.

PAIN

Pain is "an unpleasant sensory and emotional experience, associated with actual or potential tissue damage, or described in terms of such damage." There are two very important points to notice in this definition:

Pain is not just a simple physical sensation – it is also an emotional experience and should be treated as such; and

Pain isn't always associated with actual damage to the body's tissues. It may be caused by potential tissue damage, or even just feel like tissue damage even though none has actually occurred. This is referred to as neuropathic pain.

What causes the feeling of pain?

Every tissue in your body is supplied by special nerve receptors called 'nociceptors'. These are nerves which are specially designed to detect painful (or 'noxious') stimuli, for example extreme heat, mechanical damage like a pinch, or irritating chemicals. When the nociceptors detect a painful stimulus, the nerve will fire off an impulse which travels back along the nerve fibre to your spinal cord. From there, the pain message is conveyed up to the brain via a spinal neuron (nerve), travelling up through a part of the brain called the thalamus before ending in many different areas of the brain's cortex.

The parts of the brain that the pain signals are sent to are important because they affect the way we perceive pain. For example, some of the nerve fibres end in parts of the frontal lobe of the brain, which normally handles behaviour and decision-making. The pain fibres that end in the frontal lobe cause us to feel pain as an unpleasant emotional sensation, sometimes even producing fear. In contrast, the pain fibres that end in an area called the somatosensory cortex provide what we would think of as the purely 'sensory' aspects of pain, like its location and quality.

Referred pain

You may hear people talking about 'referred pain'. This means pain that originally comes from one organ or part of the body, but is felt in a different place. The commonest example is the pain of a heart attack, which may be felt in the left shoulder and down the left arm.

Referred pain occurs because of the way nerves meet up and interlink in your spinal cord. Deep structures such as the heart are supplied by different nerves from your skin. In the spinal cord, though, both of the deep and cutaneous (skin) nerves might meet up with just a single spinal nerve. This means that if the heart sends a pain signal up to the brain via that one spinal nerve, the brain can't tell whether the pain comes from the heart or from the area of skin. Because most pain signals come from the skin, and we only rarely feel pain from deep organs, the brain will interpret the signal as having come from the skin – and that is where the pain will be felt.

Pain regulation

Sensitisation

Pain Sensitisation refers to a situation where part of the pain pathway becomes over-sensitive. Sensitisation may occur after intense, repeated or prolonged stimulation of damaged tissues. When sensitisation does occur, pain fibres are more likely to be triggered in response to stimuli which would not normally be painful. This may contribute to the development of chronic pain (see below).

Gating

'Gating' is a normal regulatory mechanism which affects the way we perceive pain. The first gating mechanism is found in the spinal cord. Here, normal (non-pain) sensory fibres are linked to pain fibres in such a way that one can suppress the other. For example, after stubbing your toe (a painful stimulus), gently rubbing the skin over the toe (non-pain sensation) can reduce the feeling of pain. The non-pain sensation takes over and inhibits the transmission of the pain sensation. This mechanism is the basis of some types of pain treatment, including spinal cord stimulation.

The second gating mechanism is found in the brain. Here, emotional and psychological factors can result in the release of neurotransmitters such as endorphins. These can suppress nociceptive (pain) signals, reducing the feeling of pain.

Types of pain: Cause

Pain can be divided into a number of different types, depending on the source of the pain.

Nociceptive pain

Nociceptive pain is pain caused by damage to tissues. Tissue damage activates the nociceptive nerve fibres (see above) and pain signals are sent up through the spinal cord to the brain.

pain can be further divided into somatic pain and visceral pain, depending on the type of tissue that is damaged. The viscera are the organs of the body, so visceral pain means pain originating in an organ or hollow structure, such as the stomach or the gall bladder. Compared to the skin, these organs have a very low density of nociceptive fibres, meaning that pain from the viscera is very hard to localise, or may even be felt as referred pain. Visceral pain may be described as gnawing or aching, and may be associated with feelings of nausea.

Somatic pain refers to pain from structures other than the internal organs. This includes the bones, ligaments and tendons. This pain tends to be better localised and sharper than visceral pain.

Neuropathic pain

Neuropathic pain is a special type of pain produced by damage to part of the pain pathway. It is not associated with true tissue damage; instead, the pain pathway is 'misfiring', causing the experience of pain without actual injury. Neuropathic pain may occur after a disease such as herpes zoster infection (shingles), where damaged nociceptive nerve fibres in the skin send pain signals up to the brain even when no tissue damage is actually occurring.

Neuropathic pain is often severe, and is classically described as tingling, burning or having an electric-shock type quality. It may be associated with allodynia (severe pain on very light touch). Neuropathic pain can be highly resistant to standard pain treatments such as opiates, and antidepressant and anticonvulsant medications may be needed to help control pain.

Types of pain: Duration

PainPain can also be divided into acute pain or chronic pain.

Acute pain

Acute pain is a short-term feeling of pain felt in response to an easily identifiable cause. It might be caused by surgery, some kind of trauma, or an acute illness. The feeling of pain is acting like a sort of warning system to let you know that an injury has occurred. Acute pain lasts for less than three months.

Chronic pain

Chronic pain may begin as acute pain, but lasts longer than would normally be expected for the sort of injury that has occurred. Chronic pain may also occur when pain comes back for an unknown reason. In chronic pain syndromes, the pain may feel a lot worse than seems to fit with the injury or damage that can be seen. The link between the tissue damage and the pain is lost. Chronic pain may develop from acute pain for a number of reasons. Factors which may contribute to the development of a chronic pain syndrome include:

Presence of a chronic, painful disease such as cancer, rheumatoid arthritis, migraine headaches, fibromyalgia or diabetic neuropathy;

Damage to the sensory nerves, or painful reflex muscle contraction; or

Psychological conditions, such as depression or anxiety.

Chronic pain can be very difficult to treat, and is often frustrating for both the patient and medical professional. The optimal treatment approach should involve looking not only for the source of the pain and other physical factors, but also consideration of environmental and psychological factors which may be contributing to the pain syndrome.

Pain models

The biomedical model of pain is an older model which considers the mind and body as separate entities. This model aims to treat a single cause of pain, with little focus on emotional, psychological and other factors. It is unlikely to result in good outcomes if used to manage chronic pain.

Newer understandings of pain acknowledge that the experience of pain involves complex interactions with every part of life. This is known as the holistic model of pain. A few of the elements involved are listed below:

Physical: People with chronic pain often no longer have a single physical 'cause' for their pain. This makes treatment with medications difficult. Instead, other physical factors such as nutrition and exercise can often be more helpful.

Emotional: Anxiety, anger, guilt, blame and depression can all affect the way we experience pain. Feelings of peace and happiness can cause the release of endorphins which inhibit the feeling of pain.

Thoughts: Our thoughts and the way we think can affect messages travelling from the brain to physical structures via nerves, hormones and immune system controls.

Social: Relationships and social supports can have significant positive or negative influences on the perception of pain.

Environmental: Environments at home, or in the workplace and the broader community can also affect pain perception.

Spiritual: Addressing issues such as meaning, acceptance, hope and connection can have a positive influence on pain.

A major aim of the holistic model is to involve and empower the person with pain to help themselves.

CBD OIL FOR PAIN RELIEF?

More recently, there have been an increasing number of clinical trials to investigate modern applications of CBD. Their results have been promising which has lead to laws and legislation changing across the world. It has gotten more and more people wondering – can you use CBD for pain management and pain relief?

CBD Oil for pain – Pain types it can help with

Research has shown that cannabidiol oil can help treat numerous forms of pain in a wide variety of patients, including back pain, cancer pain, fibromyalgia pain, arthritis, and migraines. Up until recently, patients were relying on anecdotal evidence and incomplete research. Now that these clinical trials into the benefits of CBD oil is proving positive, scientists are conducting in-depth research to find definite applications of CBD.

Pain Types CBD Can Help With:

Chronic pain

Chronic pain can be utterly debilitating. It is a disease of the central nervous system where the pain goes beyond the normal timeline of healing. Chronic pain can affect numerous parts of the body. Back pain is a common form of chronic pain that some patients deal with for a long time. These can be a result of a fall or injury and manifests itself as either a sharp or dull localised pain. cannabidiol interacts with the C2 receptor in the brain which can help deal with inflammation in the body.

Cancer pains

Cancer patients must deal with an enormous amount of pain and discomfort, particularly if they opt for chemotherapy. This can cause nausea in patients, which cannabidiol has been shown to be an effective treatment for CBD as it lowers the amount of serotonin released, which reduces how often the vomiting controls in the brain are stimulated.

Multiple sclerosis

Cannabidiol has also been used to treat multiple sclerosis and other neurological diseases. This is because of its antioxidant and neuroprotective properties. This had lead to patients using cannabidiol products to try to reduce the pain and seizures associated with multiple sclerosis.

Arthritis pain

People with rheumatoid arthritis and osteoarthritis have been using CBD oil to treat their joint pain. CBD interacts with the CB2 receptor in our brains which helps reduce chronic pain and inflammation. Topical CBD oil can also be directly applied to the afflicted area to relieve joint pain which helps it to be quickly absorbed.

Migraines

It is these anti-inflammatory and pain-reducing properties that attract migraine sufferers to CBD. While it's easy to see why people with migraines turn to CBD for pain relief, definite results have yet to be proven.

Now that we know some of the many applications of cannabidiol oil you might be wondering – what's the best way to take CBD oil?

Best CBD products for pain

Just as there are many applications for CBD for pain relief, there are also scores of CBD products for pain.

NuLeaf Naturals CBD

NULEAF Naturals CBD

This CBD oil has a full spectrum of synergistic cannabinoids and terpenes. This means that it is likely to have a wider range of benefits. It is also sold in a number of strengths from 240 mg up to 4,850 mg.

CBDFX CBD Oil

This CBD oil from CBDfx is made with MCT oil. This allows for a larger amount of CBD to be absorbed by the user. It's also great for people who are on a ketogenic diet. This oil is available in 500-1500 mg doses.

Hemp Bombs CBD Oil

If you don't like the taste of CBD oil, then this might be the oil for you. They extract a CBD isolate from hemp which gives it a much milder natural flavour. It is also available in a watermelon and peppermint flavour.

CBDistilerry CBD Oil

This is a great CBD oil for the budget-conscious user. It is a full spectrum oil tincture made from non-genetically modified hemp while also being one of the most affordable oils on the market.

4 Corners CBD Oil

This CBD oil is made with the latest in filtering techniques and technology. Resulting in a CBD oil that is free from any plant material by-products.

Savage CBD Oil

If you're concerned about getting the right dosage then this might be a suitable CBD oil. It makes dosing easier as the dropper has handy measurements on it. It's also great tasting and comes in pink grapefruit, cucumber and mint, and lemon and lime flavour.

Plus CBD Oil

Looking for a non-GMO CBD oil that's also gluten-free and suitable for vegetarians? Look no further than this full-spectrum cannabidiol oil from San Diego, California.

Fab CBD Oils

Fab CBD is known for having fantastic customer service as well as brilliant products. They've got a great returns policy and brilliant pricing of shipping. Their full-spectrum CBD oil comes in five tasty flavours.

Lazarus Naturals CBD Oil

Lazarus Naturals make some of the most popular vegan and gluten-free CBD oils available. They've also designed a handy graduated dropper that allows for accurate dosing.

With so many CBD products on the market and people using them, it can seem that cannabidiol oil is a miracle cure. Are there any downsides to CBD oil? Are there any side effects?

Best ways to take CBD oil

CBD oil can be taken in a number of forms. This makes it very adaptable and should allow most users to find a method to suit their needs and lifestyle.

Different Forms of CBD

Capsules

If you're concerned about getting the correct dose every time then you might want to consider using capsules. Capsules come in exact doses that are clearly stated on the bottle. However, they do take longer to enter the bloodstream than other methods.

Tinctures

This is probably the most common method to consume CBD oil. The CBD is mixed with a carrier oil and sold in small bottles with a dropper. Tinctures are discreet and easy to use.

Edibles

CBD can also be integrated into baking and cooking. Cannabidiol oil can be added to salad dressings and easily integrated into daily life. Others enjoy CBD infused gummies, cookies and brownies.

Topicals

If you need fast-acting CBD in a precise location then you may want a topical solution. CBD infused creams, oils and balms can be directly applied to sore joints and muscles.

Vaping

If you currently vape then this it's probably best to continue vaping CBD. It works just like other vaping fluid, except this comes with all the benefits of CBD!

It seems like there are many different methods to take CBD, but what are the best CBD products for chronic pain?

CBD side effects

It's easy to see the benefits and uses of CBD, but we should all exercise some caution though. While there have been no cases of CBD-related deaths, there are some side effects to be aware of. CBD effects everyone differently so it's important to pay attention to how it affects you.

Side effects include, but not limited to:

Dry mouth

Anxiety

Weight change

Diarrhoea

Dry mouth

One of the most common side effects associated with using CBD is dry mouth or cottonmouth. This happens as CBD can affect the salivary glands. The glands are inhibited from working so the mouth is left dry and sticky. To combat this you should drink lots of water and chew on xylitol gum.

Anxiety

CBD is used by some to treat anxiety, but ironically, it can also cause anxiety in some people. It is thought that CBD can change the blood flow in areas of the brain that deal with anxiety which can increase anxiety for some people. Without further testing and research, the link between the two is still unclear.

Weight change

CBD has been known to cause both an increase and decrease in weight for users. CBD can help boost metabolism in some people which can lead to unwanted weight loss. During medical trails to investigate the relationship between CBD and epilepsy, scientists found that some patients had an increase in appetite.

Diarrhoea

Large doses of CBD have been attributed to causing diarrhoea in some people. This is caused, not by the CBD itself, but by impurities in the production process and its carrier oil.

CBD massages – Are they worth it?

The benefits of getting a massage have been well known for a long time now. They can be relaxing, therapeutic and help ease the pain. Masseuses use CBD massage oil just like regular oil on sore areas. The CBD massage oil is thought to directly affect the pain in the muscles while also acting as an anti-inflammatory. One of the main benefits of using massage oil is that you can help avoid some of the potential negatives from consuming CBD orally.

Now that we've seen the uses and benefits of CBD oil how do we choose the correct dosage?

Optimal CBD dosage for pain

As CBD affects everyone differently, it can be hard to find the correct dose that works for you. When first starting off with CBD, it is highly recommended that you speak with your doctor or professional for sound medical advice. They will recommend a dosage, to begin with.

The CBD oil dosage and it's benefits

They will use your body weight, body composition and condition being treated to estimate a good starting dose. Too low of a dose and you will see no benefit, too high and you might suffer from some side effects.

If using a CBD tincture you will need to figure out how much CBD there is per drop. This may seem daunting at first, but it's actually quite straightforward. Let's say the label on a tincture says it contains 2000 mg of CBD and the bottle has 20 ml of CBD oil in it. If one drop equals 0.05ml then you have 400 drops per 20 ml. If you have 400 drops that contain 2000 mg of CBD then 1 drop has 5 mg of CBD.

Education is one of the areas that the CBD industry and law enforcers must focus on.

When chatting with friends about CBD oil I'm sure you've had friends ask if it's legal.

Legality of CBD for pain?

Laws across the world regarding CBD and cannabis products seems to be changing quite regularly. In the EU countries like Luxembourg have stated their intent to relax laws for recreational cannabis consumption. While Canada has completely legalised cannabis and are reaping the rewards because of it.

Currently in the UK for a CBD product to be legally sold it must have a THC content level of 0.3% or less. THC is the psychoactive part of cannabis that gets you 'high'. When buying CBD products it is imperative that the labelling states how much CBD is in it and whether or not it has been tested by a third party. You can buy CBD products legally in shops and online throughout the UK.

Where to buy CBD oil

If you were to apply for CBD for pain through the NHS it is very unlikely that your request would be granted. CBD has only been prescribed in a few extreme cases. CBD users and experts hope that this will soon change. Recently, British politician's went to Canada to see the effects of cannabis legalisation. They returned with the opinion that cannabis should be legalised here in the next 10 years.

CONCLUSION

People all over the world are currently using CBD oil to treat pain. It can help with issues such as back pain, cancer pain, fibromyalgia pain, arthritis pain and migraines. Even with all these wonderful claims, it's important to realise that CBD research is still in its early days and that it can have side effects.

Once you've saught medical advice from your doctor and found the right starting dosage you can then explore all the different ways to use CBD for pain management.

cannabidiol oil can help treat numerous forms of pain in a wide variety of patients, including back pain, cancer pain, fibromyalgia pain, arthritis, and migraines. Up until recently, patients were relying on anecdotal evidence and incomplete research. Now that these clinical trials into the benefits of CBD oil is proving positive, scientists are conducting in-depth research to find definite applications of CBD.

www.ingramcontent.com/pod-product-compliance
Lightning Source LLC
Chambersburg PA
CBHW030525220526
45463CB00007B/2722